How to Design a Medical Face Mask

I0504480

A Complete Guide on How to Make Your Own Medical Face Mask At Home

Gladys Emo

Contents

Introduction

With the sudden outbreak caused by the pandemic, people are coming to terms with the need to wear a medical face mask when leaving their homes to public places like the hospital, shopping malls, religious meetings, commuting to work etc.

In some countries, the citizens have been advised by their medical practitioners to always wear face mask any time they are leaving their homes.

The fact is whether you are trying to protect yourself from germs or viruses in the public or going through a surgical operation it is pertinent to use the medical face mask as it will help to protect you and possibly prevent contracting diseases.

There are pre-made medical masks in the stores or pharmacies but unfortunately, most stores are running out of it.

As a result of the shortage, most masks most sellers have taken the advantage to inflate the price and it is now been sold on a very high scale, making it impossible for most people (especially low and average earners) to afford it.

But the good news is that you can make your medical mask at home, this can help to protect you and aid you prevent germs and any form of contamination when you are up and about doing your regular routine for the day.

This comprehensive guide has been put together to assist you in making your own making medical masks at home.

The guide will walk you through on all the different processes of making your own medical mask, the materials you will need, where you can get the materials, how you can wear your mask effectively, why you need to wear your medical mask and lots more.

So if you have been worried about where to get your medical mask, or you can't afford one, or they are not just available in your location, then you need not worry as you are on your way to making your own medical mask at home by following the steps in this text.

What is A Medical Mask?

A medical face mask otherwise known as a surgical mask is commonly used by health care experts to protect themselves and even others from the spread of airborne particulate matter, bodily build and infectious diseases.

When there's an outbreak of an infectious diseases that is easily contagious, health departments do recommend to the general public to wear medical masks to protect themselves.

Medical mask are made in a way that they are loosely fitted to cover both the nose and the mouth.

Medical mask comes in plain form, with some embellishments or decorative designs.

The Need for Medical Face Mask

One might keep on wondering about the craze for medical face mask especially with the surging demand for it amid the pandemic and might not see the need of its usage out of ignorance. The following are some of the reasons why you need to wear a medical face mask

- Wearing medical face mask gives you some level of self-protection against infectious diseases transmitted through respiratory droplets

- People with cough or respiratory infections that wear medical masks also help to eliminate or drastically reduce the spread of disease and infections
- Wearing medical mask by is a great way of to halt the continuous spread of a disease outbreak
- Medical face mask can help in filtering out some airborne particles and even some viruses that one would have come in contact with without wearing the medical face mask
- Finally, wearing medical face mask will keep your mind at peace knowing that you have an additional protection. And you would not have to panic when you find yourself in larger crowds especially during an outbreak.

A Quick Description On How To Design The Medical Mask

The designing of a medical mask is based on this mode: Note that it comes in three layers i.e. three ply and these three –ply material comes from melt-blown materials and its essence is to help filter and prevent microbes from exiting or entering the mask.

This melt-blown material is always placed in between non-woven fabric. Medical masks either have some folds or pleats. These pleats or folds are most often 3 in number, the reason for this is to enable the wearer expand the mask so as to cover from the nose to the chin area.

When it comes to using medical mask one needs to secure these three places, first the ear loop, this is the area where the string-like material is placed and it is then placed behind the ears.

Secondly behind the head which a tie- on that has four non-woven straps are tied and lastly still behind the head is the headband that is an elastic strap that is securely behind the head.

Materials Needed To Make Medical Masks

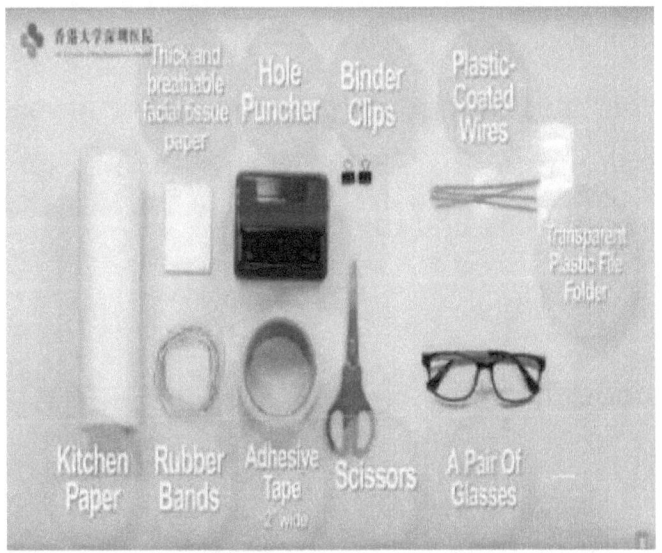

If you are thinking of making your medical mask at home, you will need the right materials to be able to get an effective medical mask.

The following are the basic materials or equipment you are likely to use but it mostly depends on what your process requires.

Note: you are not likely to use more than 3-4 materials listed below for each process. The best is to always look at the materials that are needed for each process to use, try and find out the needed materials you need per process before buying them. The following are some likely materials and their uses:

1. Paper towels

2. Rubber bands

3. Transparent plastic file holder

4. Facial tissue

5. Thick fabric

6. Elastic strips

7. Embellishments

8. Ribbons

9. Bias binding

10. Scissor

Paper towels: This is a material that can be used for medical mask because it has met the hygiene standard for medical mask material. Its fabric gaps, layout and size points makes it very effective for filtration and it can be used as the middle layer of a medical mask

Rubber bands: this a loop of rubber that you can use to hold your medical mask in place

Elastic strips; this is flexible material that is used in the making of a medical mask. It serves as a material for folding to expand the mask to cover where necessary.

Embellishments: these are decorative materials that can enhance a mask; well some people might not need a plain mask so some little embellishments can be attached to the mask to make it fashionable.

Ribbons: this is a long narrow strip used for beautification and enhancement. This material can also be added to a mask to enhance it

Bias binding: As the name implies this is a narrow strip of fabric that can be used to bind the edges of your medical mask. It is a kind of decorative feature for the mask.

Scissor; this is a material basically for the cutting of other materials used for the medical mask making process.

Adhesive tape: this will be used as sealant. It can be used in sealing off sides of the mask.

Hole puncher: used for punching holes on the medical mask for tying rubber bands or strings through it

Transparent plastic file holder: this is a transparent plastic element that can be used in on the outer layer of a medical mask, it is mostly the best choice for face protection. Using this in making a medical mask will go a long way to ward off droplets.

This plastic element is washable and can be reused if the need arises.

Facial tissue; this material is great for making medical mask. It is soft and hygienic and excellent for water absorption. It is perfect for use as the inner layer of medical mask.

After the study of facial tissue by the taskforce, we can conclude that this material is great for filtration and as such it was recommended that people should always consider using facial tissue when making medical mask at home.

This material is reusable after sterilization.

Thick fabric: this material is like cotton, it can be used on the outer layer while making a medical mask.

How to Make Medical Masks

There are different ways you can make your medical mask, some of which will be outlined below. It is up to you to choose which of the steps you prefer to use and the one you feel you can do better.

Process 1

Materials needed

Binder clips

Hole puncher

Thick and breakable facial tissue paper

Rubber bands

Kitchen paper

Adhesive tape

Scissors

Plastic coated wires

Transparent plastic file folder

The steps

Step 1; clean your materials after washing your hands thoroughly.

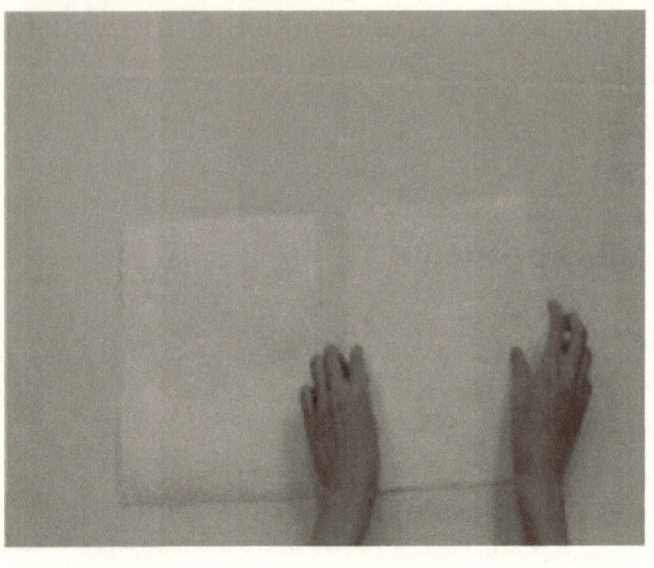

Step 2: two brands of kitchen paper can be used or you can overlap 2 pieces of the same brand to form the filter layer of the mask. (To

avoid reducing the mask filtering function don't overlap the pattern on the kitchen paper)

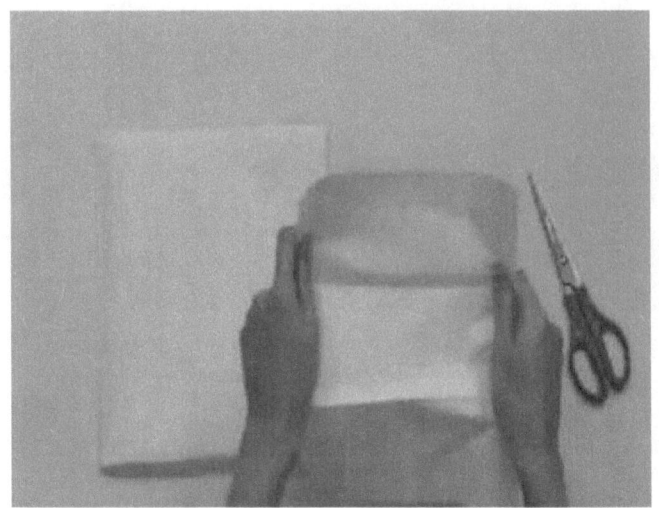

Step 3: keep a thick piece of tissue paper on top of the kitchen paper as the inner layer of your medical mask to be as the water-absorbing layer of the medical mask.

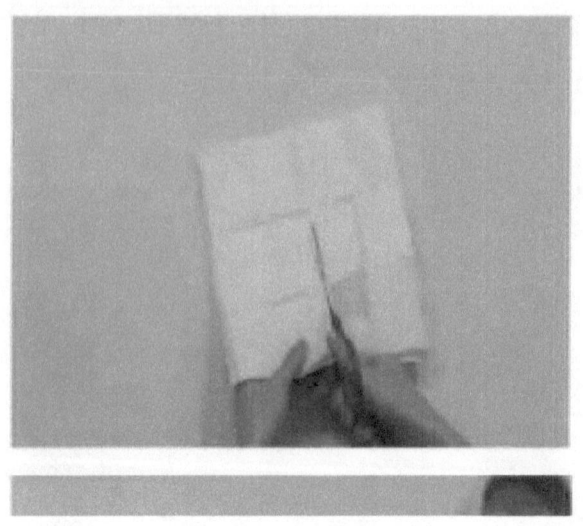

Step 4: Now, cut the stack of paper into 2, and then use the adhesive tape of about 2 inch wide to seal off the 2 sides of your product

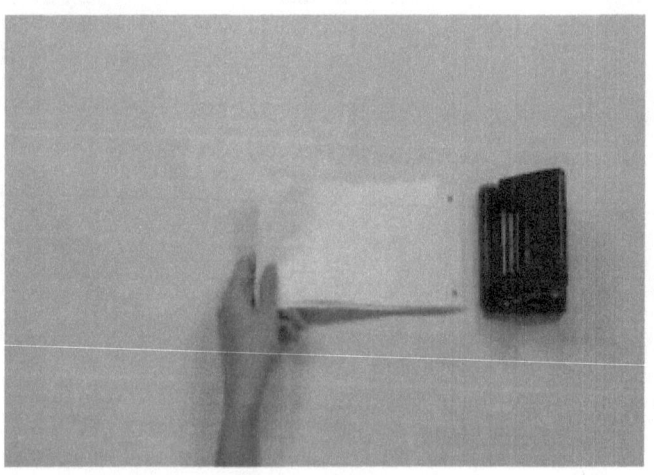

Step 5: next, punch 2 holes on each sides you have just sealed.

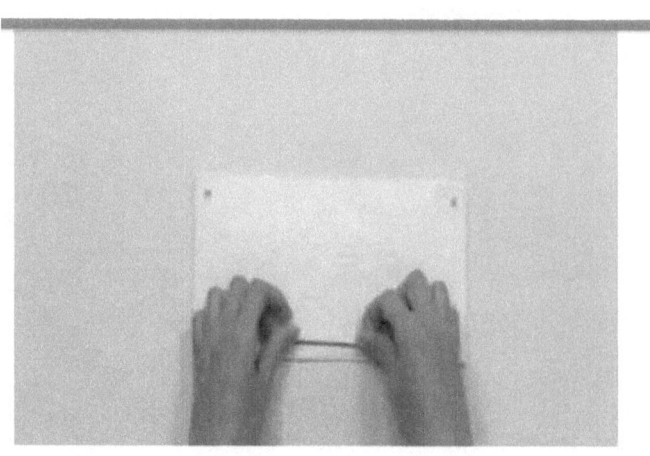

Step 6: Attach to the plastic- coated wire to a paper tape on top of the mask (for metallic wire it isn't advisable to use it without plastic coating it to prevent the risk of hurting the face or eyes.

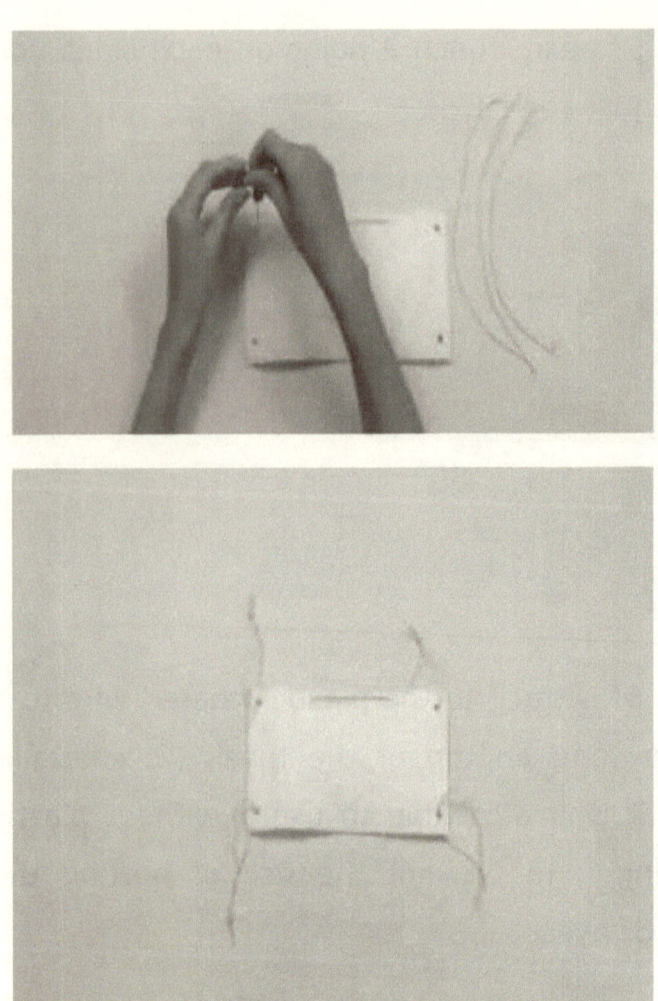

Step 7: you can now tie four strings or rubber bands through the holes on the sides of the mask's and then adjust the length (**Note:** be

18

sure the mask fit perfectly over the face. It shouldn't be too tight or too loose)

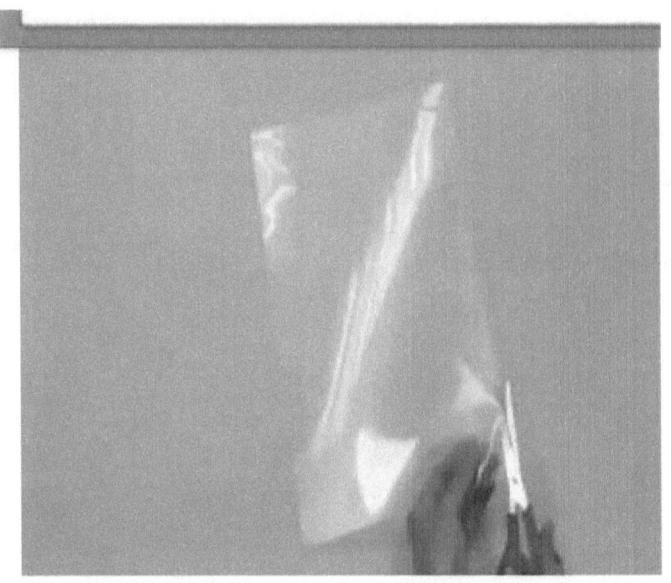

Step 8: Cut the transparent plastic file folder into 2, this will be the waterproof protection of the mask, punch 2 holes on the right corners and upper left of the plastic film and tie strings and rubber through the holes and then put the plastic film near the forehead while leaving holes on the upper part.

You can now fasten the rubber bands on the left and right hand side to fix the position.

Step 9: Alas!! You are done with making your medical mask.

Process 2

Materials needed

Thick paper

Pattern

Elastic strips

Scissor

Thick fabric

Step 1: Making a pattern for your medical mask: start by getting a piece of paper and cut out a rough medical mask shape.

You can hold it up to your face and maybe look in the mirror to see whether it is too big or too small and also check if it is too close to the eyes or down the chin?

Just keep trimming down till you get your desired shape. This will be the pattern for your medical mask.

Step 2; Place your pattern over a thick soft fabric. If you need more than 1 mask then you need to draw the pattern on the fabric as many times as you desire, for the number of masks you want. You can leave a little space though in case you make a little mistake.

Step 3: Cut half inch strips of the fabric, now fold it into half and sew it around the edges of the masks to allow the edge to be very strong and be even. Making it this way will make the seal strong to keep your breath from spreading too much.

Step 4: you need to attach the elastic strips to the medical masks to enable you loop them around your ears, securing the medical mask in place. Other ways of doing this is by getting small cords of elastic and running them through the bottom and top seams of the masks or you simply sew the length of the elastic cable to the mask at the bottom or top of the sides having the ear loops

Step 5: you have just made your first medical mask; you can try it on to ascertain if you are on the right track. If the elastic is too close to your eyes trim it to ensure it has a perfect fit.

Process 3

Materials required

60cm bias binding or ribbon

Embellishment

20x18cm fabric

Small amount of bias binding or ribbon

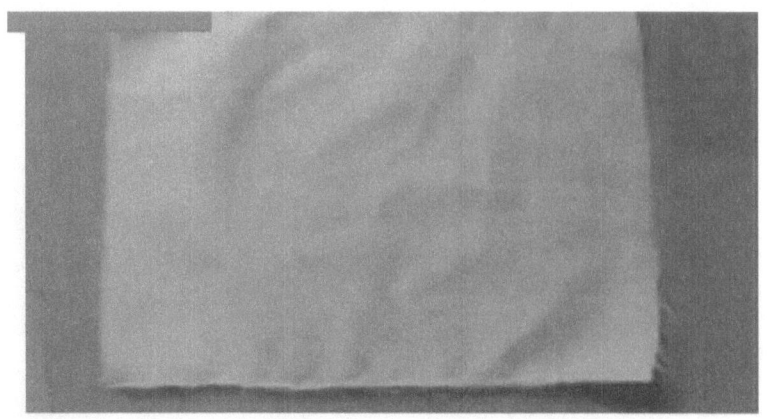

Step 1: cut a piece of fabric 20 by 18cm

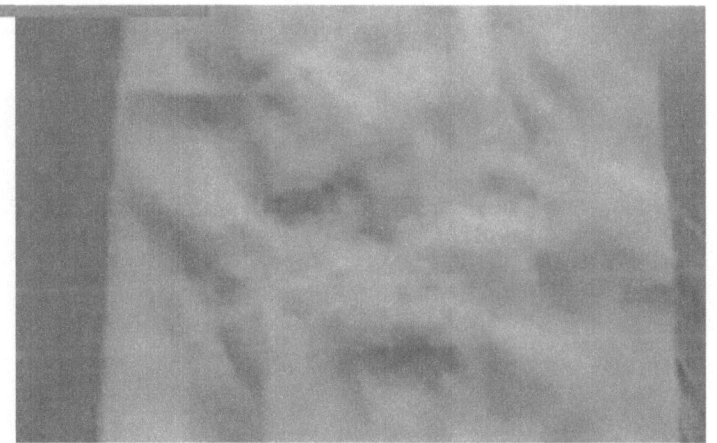

Step 2: then you can add any flat embellishments (simple bow pattern, stitch machine embroidered fun lace, ribbons or patches to the fabric

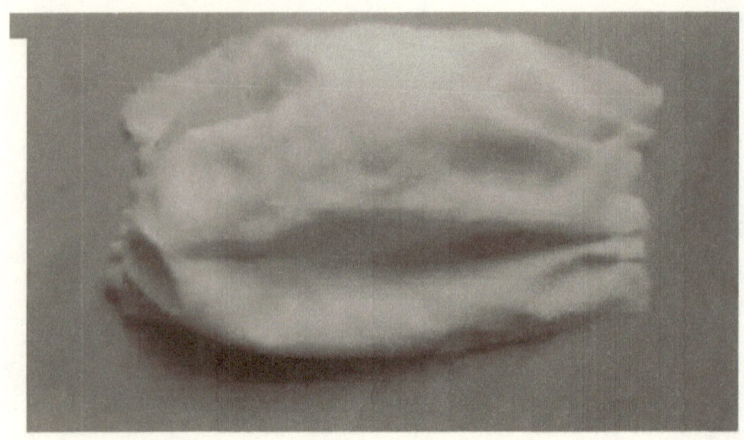

Step 3: start pleating the edges a box and 2 knife pleats to bring it down to about 9cm

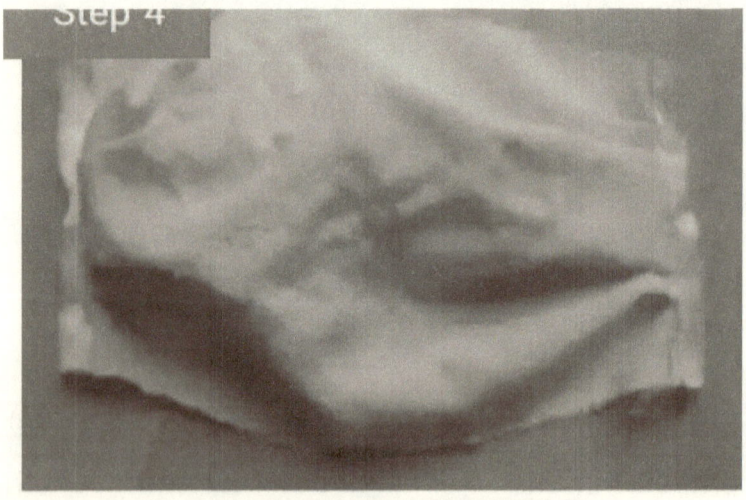

Step 4: encase the edges with bias binding or folded over ribbon

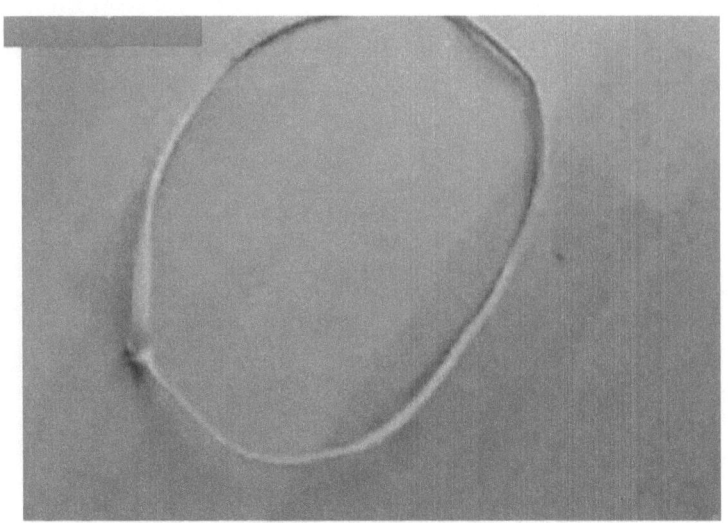

Step 5: now, sew the ends of the 60cm elastic together to make a circle

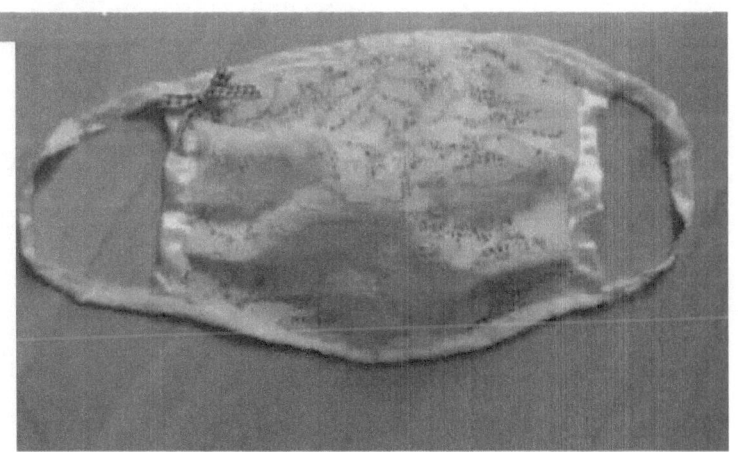

Step 6: hem the elastic into the long edges of the mask then leave 2 loops at the sides

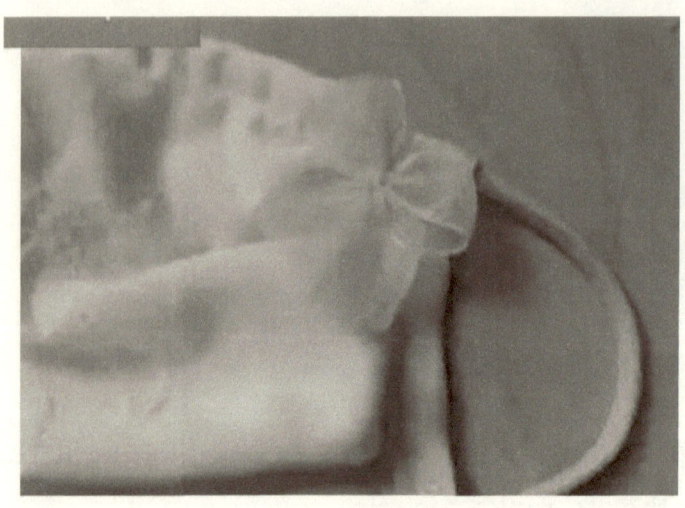

Step 7: put any extra embellishments maybe a little bow on the side just for decoration

Step 8: if you like you can encase the long edges with additional bias binding ribbon and yeah, you have a new medical mask in your hands.

Process 4

Materials required

Paper towels

Rubber bands, string or shoelaces will do

Thick fabric

Hole puncher

Steps

Step 1: take 2 or 3 squares of paper towel and lay them on top of each other, if you are using a thick fabric just cut them into equal parts and stack them on top of each other (be sure that the size you cut will be large enough to cover both your nose and mouth).

Step 2: start creating small accordion folds in the thick fabric or paper towel till the entire mask is folded into a long thin rectangle. Now, you can attach your rubber bands string or shoelaces. All of these can be achieved by you punching a hole with a hole puncher via the ends of the mask material, then you can just loop the band through stapling or gluing

Step 3; gently unfold the mask material till it is stretch out enough to cover your nose, chin and mouth

Step 4: you are almost done, check and adjust the fit of the rubber bands as you desired now

Step 5: Yippee! Your medical mask is ready

How to get the most off your medical mask

It is one thing to make and own a medical mask but the outstanding thing is getting the best of it, so now you have been able to make your own medical mask, you can use the following tips to get the most of yours.

Have a Tight Fit Mask

Do not make a loose mask if you need it to be effective for you. Medical mask shouldn't be worn for the fun of it but should meet the purpose that it was actually made for.

So make sure you make a mask that will fit snugly around your nose and mouth to help reduce numbers of foreign particles that can infiltrate the mask.

Replace It Regularly

If you are going the route of paper towels for your mask making then you need to make it enough to enable you change each regularly(the change should be once a day depending on your usage. When once you noticed your mask is wet or damp you should change it. This is necessary to do because a damp or wet mask will make you more prone to diseases and infections.

Wear your medical mask when necessary

Naturally, people that have symptoms are the ones that are suppose to wear masks in the public but those without symptoms can still wear is to wade off diseases but this should be done with caution.

The sure best is wearing them when you have yourself in a large crowd than just wearing it everywhere you go. The issue is that when medical mask are worn there's the restriction of oxygen and air flowing to the body, so to avoid an issue like this don't wear your medical mask when it isn't needed.

Cleaning of the hands

If you need your medical mask to be effective as you step out with it on your face, make sure you had thoroughly washed your hand using either alcohol based hand rub or water before making it and when you are about to wear the mask.

Have some masks in your bag for replacement

Never forget to take along with you when leaving the house whenever there's an outbreak and you are going to a public place, put some masks in a zipper storage bag that you can quickly dip your hands to get another mask for use when needed.

Avoid reusing a medical mask you made yourself

Always replace your home-made medical mask with a new one, don't reuse the old ones.

Discard a used medical mask at home in a trash can with lid and top it up with thorough washing of your hands.

Sterilize plastic file folder

To get the best from the use of plastic file folder as a material for your medical mask, always sterilize it using a diluted dishwashing, household bleach, hand wash solution or alcohol based sanitizer and rinse it with water if you need to reuse it but make sure it isn't broken or contaminated because it wouldn't be good again for use.

So just throw such away in a lidded trash can and give your hands thorough wash afterwards.

Replacing Your Mask on The Streets

You might need to replace your mask as you move about your normal routine, in this case get rid of the old one and dump it in a sealed bag before leaving it in the trash can or you can take it home for proper disposal, try not to dump it just anywhere.

Where to Use Your Medical Mask

To get the best of your homemade mask you need to know where and when to wear it.

Some places don't really require one to wear a medical mask but for places like hospital, malls, clinics, stores or clubs you should be very cautious of these high risk places but seek medical help immediately you feel the symptoms of any upper respiratory tract infection, suspected signs of infection or if you are feeling outrightly sick.

Step by step guide to effectively putting on and taking off your medical mask

Now, that you know how to get the most from your medical mask, you always need to know how you can put on and take off your mask effectively because you need to meet the purpose by which you initially thought of using a medical mask. Following the guidelines below will give you the best result ever.

Putting on a medical mask

Step 1: cleaning of your hands

This must be the first thing you do before touching your mask, wash your hands thoroughly using water and soap. Ensure you use at least 20 seconds to wash your hands under a running water before you rinse off, then use a clean paper towel to dry them.

Always endeavor to do this before discarding the paper towel in a trash can. Again, before discarding the paper towel, you can first use it on the handle of your door to open and close it before discarding the mask.

Step 2: check your mask for any defect

Before putting on your homemade mask make sure it is still in good condition as you made it. It should be devoid of holes and tears. Discard any torn mask and use other one if you notice such.

Step 3: properly orient the top of your mask

To properly have a fitted mask that will fit close to your skin as it is suppose to be. You need to make the top area or portion of the mask have a stiff edge but bendable so that you can mold it around your nose. Then you make sure that the bendable side is facing upwards before applying the mask to your face

Step 4: make sure that the proper side of your mask faces outwards

Now, the inside of most homemade medical masks made from facial tissue is always white while different colors of thick fabric can be used for the outer part. So before putting on the mask on your face make sure the white side of the mask is facing your face. So simply put, always make the inside of your mask to be on your face.

Step 5: place the mask on your face

So placing the mask on your face properly will depend on the attachment you used on your mask to enable you attach the mask to your head. So you can see the guide below for any of the material you used as an attachment.

Rubber Band: if you had used elastic bands to enable you place your mask around or over the back of your head, then just hold the mask in front of your face, pull the top band over the top of your head and place it around the crown of your head, then drag the bottom band over the top of your head and place it at the base of your skull.

Straps: if you had used straps, i.e pieces of fabric that will enable you tie your mask around the back of your head. Just go ahead pick the mask by the upper straps and tie them to the back of your head and do same to the straps below.

Ear loops: if you had made yours with ear loops, which is mostly done with an elastic material, then pick up your mask by the ear loops place 1 around the right side of the ear and the other by the other ear.

Step 6: adjusting the nose piece

Now, the mask is on your face, use your index finger to pinch the bendable area of the top edge of your mask near the bridge of your nose.

Step 7: fitting the mask under your chin and face

You are almost done with putting on your mask but before stepping out, you can adjust your mask to ascertain that it covers your face and mouth properly, same with the bottom edge which is beneath your chin.

Taking off your medical mask

Step 1: wash your hands

Well, this will depend on what you were doing with your hands prior to wanting to take your mask off. So you can either use medical gloves to remove them or wash your hands before and after taking them off.

Step 2: carefully remove the mask

Be very careful when removing your mask, it is advisable to only touch the straps, loops, bands, ties or edges when trying to get your medical mask off. Try not to touch the front portion of the mask that is contaminated already. The best bet is to remove, untie or undo ear loops, straps and bands using your hands.

Step 3: safely dispose of your mask

Remember that medical mask is meant to be worn just once.

So when once you remove the mask, dump it in the trash can, never repeat or re-use a medical mask. Better still put the used mask in a plastic bag and tie the bag before disposing it.

Step 4: clean your hands again

Once you are done disposing your mask safely, clean or wash your hands again, this is to ascertain that they remain clean and haven't been contaminated as a result of you touching the dirty mask.

Conclusion

Here you have a straightforward and simple process of making your own medical masks at home. The processes given here will assist you in producing and customizing a medical mask that will be fit for your personal use.

So if you couldn't afford the medical masks sold at the store or they are scarce in your location, you can still have them produced by yourself.

Always remember to wash your hands before and after touching your medical mask.

www.ingramcontent.com/pod-product-compliance
Lightning Source LLC
Chambersburg PA
CBHW031502210526
45463CB00003B/1045